Ginger Essential Oil

Benefits, Properties, Applications, Studies & Recipes

by Ann Sullivan

Published in USA by:

Ann Sullivan
217 N. Seacrest Blvd #9
Boynton Beach
FL 33425

© Copyright 2017

ISBN-13: ISBN-13: 978-1548104139
ISBN-10: 1548104132

Table of Contents

Introduction

What are essential oils, and how might they be used for therapeutic purposes?

Essential oils are ultra-potent oils, extracted from plants and flowers that have been utilized in medicine for centuries. Presently, they're most commonly used to supplement pharmaceutical medication, but they can also be an effective alternative to pharmaceuticals if you don't have access to them. Before you dismiss essential oils to support the body's natural defenses against injuries and illness, look at the historical evidence of the oils' therapeutic competence in practice. Your average age-old medical text will demonstrate that essential oils, herbs, and plenty of other natural ingredients have, for thousands of years, successfully enhanced immune function to meet and defeat any number of ailments and injuries. Though traditional medicine is considered "alternative" now, it was once the gold standard. And, frankly, perhaps it still should be, as these natural age-tested remedies can fortify the body's battlements against everything from simple maladies, like headaches, cuts and bruises, to serious diseases, like cancer.

Essential oils are deemed "essential," because the oils are composed of the "essence" of the plant. The difference between essential oils and other oils – like olive oil or vegetable oil, for instance – is that essential oils have high volatility and reduced fixation, which results in faster evaporation, enabling their popular use in aromatherapy.

Even at high temperatures, olive and vegetable oils don't evaporate.

Essential oils are especially necessary when it comes to a major natural or man-made disaster or some potential viral outbreak. In these types of dire situations, you may not have quick access (or any access at all) to your standard pharmaceutical supply; so, essential oils, along with other alternative medicines, will be your go-to wellness aids in the case of social collapse, viral outbreak or devastating natural disaster. When medical access is null and void, alternatives to our modern-day standard are the only chance we have to keep pathogens at bay.

You probably don't realize that you already use essential oils every day. They're in perfumes, shampoos, soaps, ointments...they're even used in furniture polish. Why are they found in so many aromatic products? Well, basically, because essential oils are super concentrated aromatic liquids, so their scent is remarkably strong. Let's put this into perspective: to steam tea, you use a few leaves of peppermint or juniper; to produce a single ounce of essential oil, five whole *pounds* of peppermint or juniper leaves are required. Some sources claim that to produce twelve pounds of essential oil would necessitate an acre of peppermint, juniper, or any other oil you're looking to produce en masse. Unlike vegetable oil, you don't often find concentrated therapeutic-grade essential oils sold by in bulk; instead the oils are often sold in easily carried small, dark bottles, perfect for your GOOD bag (Get Out Of Dodge). Which is exactly what this book is aiming to help you do –

get out of dodge with your most vital of essential oils intact, a good supply of ginger essential oil.

Why ginger, you ask? Well, to get you quickly up to speed on this most essential of oils, below we've provided a condensed synopsis of ginger, after which we'll outline in greater detail the oil's history, properties, and common therapeutic uses, so that you – the consumer – might have a better understanding of the oil's benefits and applications. We've even provided supportive remedies for pure ginger, as well as blended recipes that incorporate the valuable oil. Chapter 3 will further detail past scientific research on ginger essential oil.

Now, let's get down to it.

Essential Oil 101: the Basics of Ginger

Summary: Summary: Ginger, or Zingiber officinale, has been used for centuries in Chinese and Indian cuisine. It's traditional therapeutic uses include everything from the treatment of nausea and morning sickness to aiding circulation to soothing muscle aches.

Description: Ginger oil is commonly extracted through steam distillation. The root is most often used. The oil is typically light yellow in color, thin in consistency, and has a somewhat strong spicy and woody scent.

Uses: Beyond those applications previously mentioned, additional uses for ginger essential oil include treatment of arthritis, rheumatism, poor circulation, congestion, respiratory infections, sore throats, colds, scurvy, angina, muscle pain, motion sickness, sprains, nausea, and digestive issues, including indigestion and diarrhea. When it comes to mood and emotion, ginger helps to energize and combat fatigue.

Properties: Antioxidant, antiseptic, anticoagulant, anti-inflammatory, carminative, expectorant, analgesic, anesthetic, laxative, digestive, tonic, and stimulant properties.

Application: Dilute 1:1 with a carrier oil. You can apply topically, inhale directly, diffuse or use as a dietary supplement.

Safety Precautions: Ginger has been approved by the FDA for internal consumption and so can be used as a dietary supplement. However, if pregnant, use with caution. Also avoid if using blood thinners, as ginger is an anti-coagulant. Ginger is also photosensitive, so if used topically, avoid direct sunlight for up to 24 hours.

Fun facts: Ginger is derived from the Sanskrit word for "horn root," which is "srngaveram."

Records from ancient Greece indicate that gingerbread has been made for over 4,000 years, and the bread was used to help alleviate nausea. Ginger was also used by the Romans in their wine, because it works as an aphrodisiac.

Chapter 1 – Benefits of Ginger Essential Oil

Ginger essential oil offers several therapeutic benefits; but you may be wondering what these benefits are. In this chapter, we'll take a closer look at the history of ginger and its many uses.

Cultivation of Ginger

Originating in southern China and expanding to the Spice Islands, other Asian countries, West Africa, and the Caribbean, ginger is a flowering plant with a rhizome, ginger root, that's used as a spice. A member of the Zingiberaceae family, ginger's brothers include cardamom, turmeric, and galangal. The perennial herb grows up to three or four feet tall on average and produces yellow flowers and green leaves. The flowers are initially white and pink and are considered so aesthetically pleasing that the ginger plant is often used in landscaping in subtropical regions. The reedy plant prefers warm climates and, once the stalk withers, the rhizome is often collected, scalded, washed and scraped, to kill the root and prevent it from sprouting.

A History of Ginger

The word "ginger" is derived from the Sanskrit for "horn" and "body," "srngam" and "vera," respectively, due to the root's shape. Ginger first made its appearance in Europe in the first century AD, through spice trade with India. Currently, India continues to be the largest ginger producer, with more than 33% of global production in 2012. This is followed by China, Nepal, Nigeria, Thailand, and Indonesia.

The primary use for ginger is, of course, in cooking. As a "hot" spice, ginger's fragrance is strong, while its taste is mild. Used as an ingredient in several international cuisines, ginger is especially prevalent in Indian, Chinese, Vietnamese, Japanese, and Korean cuisine. The spice is particularly common in vegetarian, meat, and seafood dishes. In Indian cuisine, it's also used in gravies, curries, and in traditional drinks, like Masala chai. In Japan, ginger is grated or used raw in tofu and noodles dishes. The spice holds its own in bake goods as well, with gingerbread, ginger snaps, crackers, cakes and cookies all benefiting from ginger's distinct taste and aroma. This is primarily how ginger is used in Western cuisine. Beverages, too, commonly include ginger, particularly beers and ales. Ginger is often accompanied by honey and fruit in tea, and is a popular ingredient in crystallized candy or wine.

India's celebration of this spice extends to its traditional uses in Ayurvedic medicine and in the traditional folk medicine of many cultures. In India, ginger has historically served to relieve headaches and the common cold. A ginger paste is made and applied to the temples in cases of migraine. Moreover, ginger combined with black salt and lemon is mixed to alleviate nausea.

Ginger has a long history in traditional medicine, including as a carminative and stimulant often used to support issues like colic, dyspepsia, constipation, and gastroparesis. This use for digestive wellness extends to present ginger essential oil applications. Studies today indicate that ginger can provide temporary relief from nausea and vomiting.

Ginger tea has also traditionally been brewed to help support the common cold or settle the stomach. In China, for instance, boiled water, sliced ginger, and brown sugar are a regular combination to combat the common cold. In Burma, a ginger beverage is also boiled to target the flu, made from the spice and a local palm tree juice.

Moreover, the Chinese and the Philippians have long used ginger candy to suppress coughing and arthritic pain, due to inflammation, and the Indonesians create an herbal blend to help eliminate fatigue and "winds" in the blood.

In the US, ginger is primarily used for nausea, especially when it comes to morning or motion sickness. Some also target heat cramps by drinking ginger water.

Chemical Components

To generate the essential oil from ginger, the root must be steam distilled. This results in the oil's key chemical components, which are primarily zingiberene, farnesene, bisabolene, β-sesiquiphellandrene, cineol, citral, and β-phelladrene.

Main Properties of Ginger Essential Oil

Along with the properties previously mentioned in the introduction, ginger oil possesses antioxidant, antiseptic, anticoagulant, anti-inflammatory, carminative, expectorant, analgesic, anesthetic, laxative, digestive, tonic, and stimulant properties. With such a versatile range, ginger is well equipped to fight off any pathogen in the body's path.

Ginger, as mentioned, is composed of zingiberene, farnesene, bisabolene, β-sesiquiphellandrene, cineol, citral, and β-phelladrene. These components are what instill the enormously beneficial properties within ginger essential oil. We'll outline these properties below.

Antioxidant

Anything high in antioxidants – whether fruit, beans, or essential oils – is a powerful advocate for your body.

Antioxidants both protect against free radicals and repair their damage. What are free radicals? Free radicals are destructive chemicals that invade your body, produced by substances both inside and out. Some free radicals (or oxidants) form through normal bodily reactions, like inflammation, metabolism and aerobic respiration. Other free radicals form outside the body, but enter it due to exposure. These include harmful pollutants, toxins, smoking, alcohol, X-rays, and UV rays, to name a few. Although our bodies produce their own antioxidants, these often become damaged as we grow older; thus, introducing antioxidants into our bodies allows these nutrients and enzymes to assist in chemical reactions which destroy the oxidants or free radicals. Ginger essential oil is a moderate antioxidant, aiming to detox the body of free radicals that lead to disease.

Anticoagulant

As an anticoagulant, ginger essential oil combats blood clotting, which can protect against potential wellness issues like ischemic stroke, pulmonary embolism, deep vein thrombosis, and myocardial infarction.

Anti-inflammatory

External or internal inflammation can be reduced using ginger essential oil. For instance, if you or your patient has swollen fingers from arthritis or a swollen knee from a sport's injury, oral application of ginger essential oil may decrease irritation or redness, while also soothing the pain that accompanies inflammation.

Carminative

By supporting the reduction of excess gas buildup and/or removal of gas from the intestines, ginger essential oil provides relief from abdominal pain, excess sweating, and uncomfortable indigestion.

Expectorant

Throat or respiratory infections can be relieved using ginger essential oil. Acting as an expectorant, ginger breaks up and helps destroy the phlegm and mucus buildup that accompanies sinuses or respiratory infections. Inflamed throat and lungs – and, thus, coughing – can also be alleviated through the application of this oil.

Analgesic

As an analgesic, ginger essential oil supports pain relief, acting on the central nervous system to fortify the body's natural defenses against inflammation and supporting relief from pain receptor sensation.

anesthetic,

Laxative

As a laxative, ginger essential oil supplements the body's natural defenses against constipation by loosening stools and supporting bowel movements.

Digestive

By boosting the production of absorptive enzymes, the digestibility of nutrients, and the secretion of digestive juices, ginger essential oil aids the digestive tract significantly, which can make a significant impact on your overall wellness by increasing those nutrients you absorb from food.

Tonic

Ginger essential oil benefits each of the body's systems, whether nervous, digestive, respiratory or excretory, making it an unbeatable general tonic. The oil also supports the immune system by helping the body absorb nutrients.

Stimulant

Stimulants are often referred to as "uppers." This is because they produce mental or physical improvements or temporary enhancements of your bodily functions. For instance, you may grow more alert and awake or quicker on your feet after using a stimulant. Ginger essential oil can provide this temporary boost in mental and physical function, especially when it comes to the immune system.

Common Therapeutic Uses

Traditionally used to enhance the body's defenses against nausea and digestive issues, ginger essential oil remains a significant digestive stimulant, protecting against several conditions, like nausea and constipation. Ginger essential oil supports overall wellness, while relieving inflammation and pain. Let's take a closer look at the common uses for this oil.

Immune System Booster

Ginger is a superb immune system support which boosts circulation and increases white blood cell count. The oil is akin to an immune shield braced to fight off inflammatory strains that attack the immune system. With such strong armor, this immune stimulant will ensure that your body is better prepared to protect against deadly infections.

Digestion

As a digestive aid, ginger essential oil's collective properties stimulate digestive enzyme secretion which serves to support issues like constipation, upset stomach, flatulence, indigestion, heartburn, colic, diarrhea, dyspepsia, and stomach cramps. Moreover, research shows that it can effectively combat nausea and vomiting, due to motion or morning sickness. As ginger is often used as a spice, particularly in Indian dishes, the digestive properties are coupled with an enrichment of culinary flavor.

Cardiovascular Wellness

Cardiovascular wellness can be maintained through the abundance of vitamins and minerals found in ginger essential oil, which include calcium, magnesium, and iron. The oil contains dietary fiber as well, which along with its other contents, helps to reduce bad cholesterol (LDL) and boost good cholesterol (HDL), resulting in better cardiovascular wellness. The oil's antioxidant properties and its ability to facilitate the dissolution of cholesterol that accumulates in arteries will also support cardiovascular issues, like heart disease or atherosclerosis.

Women's Wellness

Ginger can significantly benefit women at any age or in any condition, as it helps relieve cramps when it comes to painful periods and eliminate nausea due to morning sickness. If you commonly experience painful or irregular periods that impact your daily life, a ginger application can both help relieve the pain and uplift the spirit.

Respiratory Issues

As an anti-inflammatory, ginger essential oil calms coughing by opening the airways. Bronchitis, congestion, asthma, sinusitis, cough, and other respiratory issues can be supported with ginger essential oil, as the oil is an expectorant that promotes a healthy respiratory tract, soothes the throat, and clears nasal passages.

Stress Disorders

Whether it be physical stress or mental stress, ginger's aroma, in conjunction with its therapeutic properties, enable its use in the support of stress disorders, like upset nerves, anxiety, melancholy, and depression. It can help soothe mental fatigue and refresh cognitive function.

Headache & Nausea

One of ginger's simplest but most effective therapeutic uses is to relieve headache pain and nausea. With a simple rub of the diluted oil on the temples and forehead, the calming, soothing properties of ginger quickly eliminate the strongest and most stubborn of headaches, as both the refreshing scent and the oil's anti-inflammatory and analgesic properties help to alleviate tension. You can also simply inhale the scent from the bottle to soothe both headaches and nausea from motion sickness.

Safety Precautions & Common Applications

Safety

Certain adverse effects may evolve when using pure essential oils. Some essential oils should not be used when pregnant, for example, as they may cause miscarriage. Allergic reactions, too, may occur, especially when applied topically. Always administer an allergy test before committing fully to topical application. When used with other medications, essential oils may react negatively. If you are on any current prescription medications or have a chronic illness, such as high blood pressure, epilepsy or liver disease, then researching the effects of essential oils against your own personal medical history will eliminate any potentially problematic issues.

Ginger has been approved by the FDA for internal consumption and so can be used as a dietary supplement. Ginger is photosensitive, so if used topically, avoid direct sunlight for up to 24 hours. Ginger also an anti-coagulant, so if you're using it alongside blood thinners, their effects will be enhanced. If you are pregnant, use with caution and at the discretion of your physician. If you have sensitive skin, dilute heavily and test before extensive use. Otherwise, dilute 1:1 with a carrier oil. You can apply topically, diffuse or use as a dietary supplement.

Blends

Oftentimes, essential oils are manufactured as blends of several pure oils. For instance, the Protective Blend of certain brands is a mix of cinnamon, clove, rosemary, and eucalyptus. This blend can be used to boost the immune system to help support colds, viruses and flus. The downside to blends is that the more oils added to the mix, the higher the probability your patient may react negatively to the blend if he/she is prone to allergies. There is also the possibility of phototoxicity when working with blends, particularly if they include citrus oils. Be sure to read your labels before administering.

Regardless of these possible effects, essential oils are a viable option for supporting several conditions. Those looking to support or maintain their own personal wellness, or that of their families', should become educated on the uses of essential oils, their natural remedies and the methods of application. Only then can you begin building your kit of essential oils for survival.

Chapter 2 – Recipes for Ginger Essential Oil

In this chapter, we'll offer various recipes for ginger essential oil, both for pure ginger applications and blends. For pure applications, we've provided the appropriate dosage and method of administration to support specific ailments, from angina to vertigo. When it comes to blends, herbalists and aromatherapists often combine ginger essential oil with ylang ylang, lemon, orange, cedarwood, rosewood, lime, bergamot, eucalyptus, sandalwood, frankincense, patchouli, geranium, and rosemary. We'll offer some fantastic blending options in the second half of this chapter.

Pure Applications

Angina

To relieve angina and stress while stimulating the circulatory system, dilute ginger essential oil in a 1:1 ratio with a carrier oil and apply topically, massaging over the heart up to three times daily.

Appetite Stimulant

If grief, stress, illness, or depression causes you to experience appetite loss, diffuse ginger essential oil throughout the home.

Chills

If you're feeling the chills, dilute ginger essential oil in a 1:1 ratio with a carrier oil and apply topically, massaging the oil into the soles of the feet.

Club Foot

Alleviate the pain and inflammation of a club foot by diluting ginger essential oil in a 1:1 ratio with a carrier oil; then apply topically, massaging into the affected area.

Colds

Combat the common cold by diffusing ginger essential oil throughout the home. You can also apply topically by diluting the oil in a 1:1 ratio with a carrier oil and massaging into the chest and the soles of the feet.

Cooking

You can use ginger essential oil in cooking, as it's generally regarded as safe by the FDA. One drop (or less) to begin with; add more to taste. A little oil goes a long way. Ginger goes great in soup or when combined with soy sauce for a stir-fry.

Courage

To enhance courage or bravery, place a drop of ginger essential oil into your hands, rub your palms together, cup them over your nose, and breathe deeply in and out for several minutes. You may also choose to dilute ginger essential oil in a 1:1 ratio with a carrier oil and apply topically, massaging into the upper and lower abdomen and over the solar plexus. Use daily for the best results.

Cramps

Alleviate menstrual, intestinal, or abdominal cramps by diluting ginger essential oil in a 1:1 ratio with a carrier oil and applying topically. Massage into the lower abdomen and back and into the reflex points of the feet.

Diarrhea

If you're experiencing diarrhea, ginger essential oil is

the answer. Apply topically by diluting the oil in a 1:1 ratio with a carrier oil and massaging it into the abdomen in a counterclockwise motion, or place a drop of the oil in your drinking water or your meals throughout the day.

Empower

If you're experiencing self-doubt and need to boost trust and empowerment within, pour a drop of ginger essential oil into your hands, rub your palms together, cup them over your nose, and breathe deeply in and out for several minutes. You can also apply topically, diluting ginger essential oil in a 1:1 ratio with a carrier oil and massaging into the lower abdomen.

Flatulence

Relieve gas by diluting ginger essential oil in a 1:1 ratio with a carrier oil and massaging into the abdomen in a clockwise motion. You can also place a drop in a glass of water and take orally.

Immune Stimulant

Give your immune system a leg up by regularly diffusing ginger essential oil throughout your home, especially during cold and flu season. Alternatively, you can add a couple drops to your bathwater or dilute in a 1:1 ratio with a carrier oil and apply topically, massaging the oil into the feet. If you'd prefer the steam method, steam two drops of ginger essential oil in a pan of water, remove the steaming pan from the stove, pour into a bowl, place a towel over your head and inhale. If you don't feel it's done its job the first time, you can reheat that same water and use it once more without adding more oil.

Impotency Support

Ginger essential oil enhances circulation and relaxes the muscles. The oil is also said to aid in issues of impotency. To administer, dilute ginger essential oil in a 1:1 ratio with a carrier oil and massage into the reflex points of the feet.

Indigestion

Ginger aids the digestive tract and can be taken orally or topically. Place a drop into your drinking water for internal administration or dilute the oil in a 1:1 ratio with a carrier oil and apply topically to the abdomen in a clockwise motion and into the reflex points of the feet. You can also diffuse throughout the home.

Libido

Ginger has long been used to stimulate the libido. Diffuse regularly or dilute ginger essential oil in a 1:1 ratio with a carrier oil and apply topically, massaging into the lower stomach and the soles of the feet.

Memory

Stimulate the memory by steaming two drops of ginger

essential oil in a pan of water. Then remove the steaming pan from the stove, pour into a bowl, place a towel over your head and inhale. If you don't feel it's done its job the first time, you can reheat that same water and use it once more without adding more oil. You can also diffuse the oil wherever you study or work. Additionally, try inhaling directly, adding a few drops to bathwater, or diluting in a 1:1 ratio with a carrier oil and massaging into the base of the toes.

Motion Sickness

To stave off or relieve motion sickness, apply a single drop of ginger essential oil to car seats. You can also place a drop on a piece of cloth or on the shirt collar to be inhaled whenever you feel nausea coming on.

Motivation

Give yourself a motivational leg up by diffusing throughout your home or car. You can also place a drop on your shirt sleeve or inhale directly whenever you're feeling stressed. To apply topically, dilute ginger essential oil in a 1:1 ratio with a carrier oil and massage over the solar plexus.

Muscle Aches

To relieve sore muscles, dilute ginger essential oil in a 1:1 ratio with a carrier oil and massage the solution into the affected area, toward the heart.

Nausea

Stave off or relieve nausea by applying a single drop to a piece of cloth or on the shirt collar to be inhaled when feeling nauseous. You can also diffuse or topically apply ginger essential oil, diluted in a 1:1 ratio with a carrier oil, massaging the solution into the abdomen. You can also take internally. Place a drop in your drinking water and drink slowly.

Pelvic Pain Syndrome

To relieve the pain of pelvic pain syndrome, dilute ginger essential oil in a 1:1 ratio with a carrier oil and apply topically, massaging into the affected area up to three times daily.

Rheumatic Fever

Combat the pain and inflammation of rheumatism by diluting ginger essential oil in a 1:1 ratio with a carrier oil; then apply topically, massaging the oil into the affected area. You can also simply diffuse or use the steam method. Steam two drops of the oil in a pan of water, remove the steaming pan from the stove, pour into a bowl, place a towel over your head and inhale. If you don't feel it's done its job the first time, you can reheat that same water and use it once more without adding more oil.

Rheumatoid Arthritis

Similarly, to the above recommendation, dilute ginger essential oil in a 1:1 ratio with a carrier oil and apply topically, massaging the oil into the joints, to relieve pain and inflammation.

Tonsillitis

Eliminate tonsillitis by diluting ginger essential oil in a 1:1 ratio with a carrier oil and applying topically in a full-body massage. You can also diffuse throughout the home or combine the oil with sea salts and warm water for a gargling solution.

Vertigo

Combat vertigo and maintain balance by ginger essential oil throughout the home. You can also pour a drop into your hands, rub your palms together, cup them over your nose, and breathe deeply for thirty seconds. To apply topically, dilute ginger essential oil in a 1:1 ratio with a carrier oil and massage into the back of the neck and into the reflex points of the feet.

Vomiting

To help stave off vomiting, place a drop of ginger essential oil in your drinking water. You can apply topically, diluting the oil in a 1:1 ratio with a carrier oil, massaging it into the abdomen and into the reflex points of the feet. You can also inhale directly or diffuse throughout the home.

Blends

Ankle Swelling Relief

Ingredients

- 3 drops Ginger Essential Oil
- 3 drops Lemon Essential Oil
- 3 drops Geranium Essential Oil
- 3 drops Lavender Essential Oil
- 1 Tbsp. Grapeseed Oil

Directions

To reduce ankle swelling during pregnancy, combine all ingredients and apply directly to the affected area several times each day, massaging the feet and ankles upwards, toward the heart.

Aphrodisiac Massage Blend

Ingredients

- 1 drop Ginger Essential Oil
- 1 drop Clove Essential Oil
- 2 drops Cinnamon Essential Oil
- 2 drops Peppermint Essential Oil
- 3 drops Jasmine Essential Oil
- 3 drops Vanilla Absolute
- 2 ounces Carrier Oil

Directions

To stimulate sexual arousal for men and women, combine all ingredients in a small bowl, blending well. Apply in a full body massage or into the reflex points (*caution: cinnamon essential oil is hot and may irritate sensitive skin; if you are prone to skin irritation, increase the amount of carrier oil).

Aphrodisiac Massage Blend II

Ingredients

- 2 drops Black Pepper Essential Oil
- 2 drops Ginger Essential Oil
- 3 drops Wild Orange Essential Oil
- 3 drops Rosemary Essential Oil
- 4 drops Ylang Ylang Essential Oil
- 4 drops Bergamot Essential Oil
- 4 drops Sandalwood Essential Oil
- 4 ounces Carrier Oil (fractionated coconut oil recommended)

Directions

To stimulate sexual arousal for men and women, combine all ingredients in a small bowl, blending well. Apply in a full body massage or into the reflex points. Store in a glass bottle.

Appetite Stimulant

Ingredients

- 8 drops Clary Sage Essential Oil
- 6 drops Coriander Essential Oil
- 4 drops Black Pepper Essential oil
- 3 drops Ginger Essential Oil
- 2 drops Peppermint Essential Oil

Directions

To help stimulate appetite, diffuse throughout the home or pour the blend into your inhalant to use throughout the day. Those who have recently been ill or going through chemotherapy can boost their appetite through frequent inhalation.

Arthritic Massage Oil

Ingredients

- 2 drops Black Pepper Essential Oil
- 2 drops Ginger Essential Oil
- 3 drops Coriander Essential Oil
- 4 drops Helichrysum Essential Oil
- 5 drops Roman Chamomile Essential Oil
- 2 ounces Carrier Oil

Directions

To relieve arthritic pain, combine all ingredients in a small bowl, blending well. Apply topically, massaging the oil into the affected area. Use as needed.

Arthritic Massage Oil II

Ingredients

- 1 drop Black Pepper Essential Oil
- 1 drop Ginger Essential Oil
- 3 drops Rosemary Essential Oil
- 3 drops Coriander Essential Oil
- 4 drops Marjoram Essential Oil
- 6 drops Roman Chamomile Essential Oil
- 2 ounces Carrier Oil

Directions

To relieve arthritic pain, combine all ingredients in a small bowl, blending well. Apply topically, massaging the oil into the affected area. Use as needed.

Arthritic Massage Oil III

Ingredients

- 1 drop Ginger Essential Oil
- 2 drops Cilantro Essential Oil
- 3 drops Cypress Essential Oil
- 2 Tbsps. Carrier Oil

Directions

Relieve arthritic pain by combining all ingredients in a small container. Tighten the lid and shake well. Apply topically, massaging into arthritic wrists or knees whenever you're in need of pain relief.

Chills & Colds Warming Bath Blend

Ingredients

- 2 drops Ginger Essential Oil
- 2 drops Benzoin Essential Oil
- 2 drops Wild Orange Essential Oil
- 1 Tbsp. Grapeseed Oil

Directions

For a bath that warms you to the bones, add all ingredients to your bathwater and stir to disperse. Then inhale deeply while you soak for 20 minutes, but avoid getting water in your eyes, as it may sting. Great during cold season.

Cold Diffusion Blend

Ingredients

- 4 drops Ginger Essential Oil
- 6 drops Basil Essential Oil
- 6 drops Rosewood Essential Oil
- 10 drops Juniper Berry Essential Oil
- 10 drops Eucalyptus Essential Oil
- 10 drops Pine Essential Oil
- 20 drops Orange Essential Oil
- 15 mL Carrier Oil

Directions

In a small jar or container, mix all ingredients until well combined. Diffuse several drops of the blend as needed, especially during cold and flu season or whenever your immune system feels weakened.

Concentration

Ingredients

- 3 drops Black Pepper Essential Oil
- 3 drops Ginger Essential Oil
- 3 drops Cardamom Essential Oil
- 3 drops Basil Essential Oil

Directions

To help focus concentration and be present, diffuse throughout the bedroom.

Constipation/Diarrhea

Ingredients

- 2 drops Fennel Essential Oil
- 2 drops Peppermint Essential Oil
- 1 drop Ginger Essential Oil

Directions

To relieve constipation or diarrhea, place all ingredients into a "00" capsule and ingest every three hours until the issue is resolved.

Crave-Curbing Blend

Ingredients

- 1 drop Ginger Essential Oil
- 1 drop Peppermint Essential Oil
- 2 drops Lemon Essential Oil
- 5 drops Mandarin Essential Oil
- 2-ounce Jojoba or Almond Oil

Directions

In a small bowl or container, mix all ingredients until well combined. To relieve cravings, apply topically, massaging into the reflex points of the feet. You may also inhale directly or diffuse (without the carrier oil).

Digestive Support

Ingredients

- 1 drop Blue Tansy
- 2 drops Fennel Essential Oil
- 2 drops Ginger Essential Oil
- 3 drops Tarragon Essential Oil
- 8 drops Rosemary Essential Oil
- 10 drops Anise Essential Oil
- 8 ounces Carrier Oil

Directions

In a small jar or container, mix all ingredients until well combined. For digestive support, use as needed. Apply topically, massaging over the abdomen and into the reflex points of the feet. Mix well before each use.

Erectile Dysfunction Blend

Ingredients

- 1 drop Jasmine Essential Oil
- 1 drop Black Pepper Essential Oil
- 1 drop Sandalwood Essential Oil
- 1 drop Nutmeg Essential Oil
- 1 drop Ginger Essential Oil
- 1 Tbsp. Sweet Almond Oil

Directions

The issue of erectile dysfunction is often influenced by poor blood flow. The oils in this blend enhance blood flow and circulation. To administer, you may apply to a warm compress or massage into the lower back. You can also add the oils (no need for the carrier oil) to a hot bath.

Fallen Arches

Ingredients

- 5 drops Black Pepper Essential Oil
- 5 drops Clary Sage Essential Oil
- 10 drops Ginger Essential Oil
- 10 drops Rosemary Essential Oil
- 2 Tsp Carrier Oil

Directions

To relieve the stress of fallen arches, combine all ingredients in a small bowl, blending well. Apply to the instep of the foot, massaging toward the heel.

Fatigue

Ingredients

- 1 drops Ginger Essential Oil
- 2 drops Clary Sage Essential Oil
- 2 drops Sandalwood Essential Oil
- 2 drops Cilantro Essential Oil
- 3 drops Frankincense Essential Oil
- ½ Tbsp. Carrier Oil

Directions

To combat fatigue, combine all ingredients in a small bowl or container, blending well. Apply topically to the forearms and the back of the neck, inhaling the scent deeply.

Gluten Intolerance

Ingredients

- 1 drop Cinnamon Bark Essential Oil
- 2 drops Grapefruit Essential Oil
- 2 drops Ginger Essential Oil
- 2 drops Lemon Essential Oil

Instructions

To help strengthen the body's natural defenses against gluten intolerance, place all ingredients into a "00" capsule, and ingest 1 capsule a day.

Headache Relief

Ingredients

- 5 drops Clove Essential Oil
- 6 drops Ginger Essential Oil
- 9 drops Peppermint Essential Oil
- 9 drops Wintergreen Essential Oil
- 4 tsps. Carrier Oil

Directions

To relieve headaches, combine all ingredients in a small bowl, blending well. Apply to the temples, forehead, back of the neck, the reflex points, or in a full body massage.

Immune-Boosting Spray

Ingredients

- 4 ounces Distilled Water
- 60 drops Ginger Root Essential Oil
- 20 drops Cinnamon Bark Essential Oil

Directions

Combine all ingredients in a dark colored glass spray bottle and, during cold and flu season or if there's illness in the house, spray in all rooms to stimulate the immune system.

Immune-Boosting Massage

Ingredients

- 2 drops Frankincense Essential Oil
- 2 drops Ginger Essential Oil
- 2 drops German Chamomile Essential Oil
- 1 drop Cinnamon Essential Oil
- 2 ounces Carrier Oil

Directions

In a small jar or container, mix all ingredients until well combined. Apply topically during cold and flu season, massaging into the reflex points of the feet or in a full-body massage.

Morning Sickness Relief

Ingredients

- 1 drop Lemon Essential Oil
- 1 drop Ginger Essential Oil
- 1 tsp Honey
- 8 ounces Drinking Water

Directions

To combat morning sickness, mix all ingredients until well combined and drink.

Motion Sickness

Ingredients

- 2 drops Orange Essential Oil
- 2 drops Ginger Essential Oil
- 2 drops Roman Chamomile Essential Oil

Directions

To relieve nausea and vomiting while traveling, add all ingredients to a tissue or cloth and inhale whenever you feel motion sickness coming on, breathing deeply in and out.

Relaxing Diffusion Blend

Ingredients

- 2 drops Sandalwood Essential Oil
- 4 drops Ginger Essential Oil
- 6 drops Lime Essential Oil
- 6 drops Grapefruit Essential Oil
- 6 drops Bergamot Essential Oil

Directions

In a small jar or container, mix all ingredients until well combined. Diffuse several drops of the blend as needed, especially during stressful times or when you want to unwind.

Warming Massage Blend

Ingredients

- 2 drops Ginger Essential Oil
- 3 drops Black Pepper Essential Oil
- 5 drops Sandalwood Essential Oil
- 15 drops Ylang Ylang Essential Oil
- 15 mL Carrier Oil

Directions

In a small bowl or container, mix all ingredients until well combined. Warm slightly then to help relax and relieve sore muscles and stimulate libido, apply in a full-body massage.

Chapter 3 – Ginger Essential Oil Studies

Many studies have been done on essential oils to uncover and prove their therapeutic qualities. In the case of the great number of ginger studies, many of the properties attributed to the essential oil (noted in this book and elsewhere) are quite often validated through the research from accredited universities and published by reputable scientific journals. In this chapter, we'll discuss a small portion of these studies. It's important to note that our knowledge of essential oils is constantly evolving. Keep up with any recent research, as it may turn up even further valuable uses for these miracle oils.

Study 1 – Anticancer

In this study published by the *Asian Pacific Journal of Cancer Prevention*, the anticancer activities of ginger essential oil were examined, with the following results: "Patients with colorectal cancer are usually treated with chemotherapy, which reduces the number of blood cells, especially white blood cells, and consequently increases the risk of infections. Some research studies have reported that aromatherapy massage affects the immune system and improves immune function by, for example, increasing the numbers of natural killer cells and peripheral blood lymphocytes...The objectives of this study were to determine whether the use of aromatherapy with light Thai massage in patients with colorectal cancer, who have received chemotherapy, can result in improvement of the cellular immunity and reduce the severity of the common symptoms of side effects...Aromatherapy with light Thai massage can be beneficial for the immune systems of cancer patients who are undergoing chemotherapy by increasing the number of lymphocytes and can help to reduce the severity of common symptoms."

Colorectal cancer occurs in the large intestine often in the rectum or colorectal. Abnormal cell growth in these regions invade and often spread to other parts of the body. The cancer is more common in men than women, and heredity rarely plays a part in the diagnosis. Colorectal cancer regularly first grows as a benign tumor or polyp before becoming cancerous. If caught early and confined to the colorectal, colorectal cancer can be cured, but if the cancer has spread, the outcome is rarely curable. Worldwide, colorectal cancer diagnoses make up 10% of all cancer cases and is the third most common cancer type. In the US, the five-year survival rate of the disease is 65%. The stats for 2012 indicate that 1.4 million new cases were diagnosed, and there were 694,000 died from the cancer.

Colorectal cancer patients receive chemotherapy treatment, which increases the risk of infections due to the reduction in the number of blood cells, specifically white blood cells. This study's objective was to identify the biological mechanisms by which aromatherapy massage affects and improves immune function, as has previously been reported. Moreover, the study evaluated whether aromatherapy massage boosted the numbers of peripheral blood lymphocytes and natural killer cells.

The study examined 66 patients with colorectal cancer. Over the period of a week, the patients in the experimental group received three massage sessions with ginger and coconut oil over a 1-week period and the levels of lymphocytes (a type of white blood cell found in the lymph), white blood cells, neutrophils, CD4 and CD8 cells and the CD4/CD8 ratio were assessed. What the study found was that the average lymphocyte count was significantly higher (P=0.04) in the treatment group when compared with the controls after the ginger massage treatment. The results indicated that the combination of ginger essential oil and Thai massage has potential to improve lymphocyte numbers by 11%, while also reducing stress, pain and fatigue, all of which are beneficial to immune system function.

These results demonstrate the efficacy of using ginger

essential oil in combination with Thai massage to support immune system function in the case of colorectal cancer or to boost general immune system function.

Reference

http://www.ncbi.nlm.nih.gov/pubmed/23886205]

http://www.apocpcontrol.org/page/apjcp_issues_view.php?sid=Entrez:PubMed&id=pmid:23886205&key=2013.14.6.3903]

Study 2 – Nausea

In this study available on PubMed, the effects of ginger essential oil on postoperative nausea were examined, with the following results: "Postoperative nausea (PON) is a common complication of anesthesia and surgery. Antiemetic medication for higher-risk patients may reduce but does not reliably prevent PON. We examined aromatherapy as a treatment for patients experiencing PON after ambulatory surgery. Our primary hypothesis was that in comparison with inhaling a placebo, PON will be reduced significantly by aromatherapy with (1) essential oil of ginger, (2) a blend of essential oils of ginger, spearmint, peppermint, and cardamom, or (3) isopropyl alcohol. Our secondary hypothesis was that the effectiveness of aromatherapy will depend upon the agent used...The hypothesis that aromatherapy would be effective as a treatment for PON was supported. Based on our results, future research further evaluating aromatherapy is warranted. Aromatherapy is promising as an inexpensive, noninvasive treatment for PON that can be administered and controlled by patients as needed."

This study aimed to assess the efficacy of ginger essential oil on its own, as well as a blend of essential oils that combined cardamom, ginger, spearmint and peppermint, on nausea postanesthesia care. 301 subjects were analyzed, and were asked to provide a description of their level of nausea on a 0-3 scale, after which they were provided either the blend, ginger on its own, or isopropyl alcohol. The study found that the reduction in the level of nausea significantly decreased when provided the blend (P < 0.001) and ginger (P = 0.002), and the amount of antiemetic medications requested afterward decreased significantly as well. This demonstrates the potential for ginger essential oil, administered either solo or in a blend, as an antidote to nausea.

Reference
http://www.ncbi.nlm.nih.gov/pubmed/22392970]

Study 3 – Anti-inflammatory Properties

In this study available on PubMed, the anti-inflammatory effects of ginger essential oil were examined, with the following results: "The pro-inflammatory chemokine interleukin-8 is increased in asthmatic patients. Traditionally, ginger is used as an anti-inflammatory drug. An extract and several compounds of Zingiber officinale (ginger) were tested in human bronchial epithelial cells...Our results suggest that distinct ginger compounds could be used as anti-inflammatory drugs in respiratory infections."

The study's objective was to evaluate ginger essential oil's anti-inflammatory effects on bronchial epithelial cells, with regards to chemokine interleukin-8, which is a signaling protein created by cells – in this case bronchial epithelial cells – that is often associated with inflammation. The results showed that ginger essential oil – in the form of an oily extract containing 25% total pungent compounds, ginger volatile oil, ar-curcumene and α-pinene – reduced interleukin-8 secretion, indicating that this ability to shut down the secretion of the inflammatory chemokine is the mechanism by which ginger essential oil is effective in regards to respiratory infections and general respiratory support.

Reference
http://www.ncbi.nlm.nih.gov/pubmed/21698672]

Study 4 – Antioxidant, Anti-inflammatory & Anti-proliferative Properties

In this study published in *PLOS ONE*, the activities of various essential oils on prostate cancer were examined, with the following results: "This research highlights the chemical composition, antioxidant, anti-inflammatory and anti-proliferative activities of essential oils from leaves of… Zingiber officinale… Anti-inflammatory properties were evaluated by measuring the inhibition of lipoxygenase activity and essential oil of Z. officinale was the most active… Altogether these results justify the use of these plants in traditional medicine in Burkina Faso and open a new field of investigation in the characterization of the molecules involved in anti-proliferative processes."

The dozens of essential oils examined in this study demonstrated activity against several cancerous cell lines, as well as antioxidant and anti-inflammatory properties. Of those oils tested, the essential oils of chickweed and honeysuckle were the most active against the LNCaP and PC-3 cell lines. Although these two essential oils are not popularly commercially produced, several the other oils tested exhibited anti-cancer activity, as well. Moreover, the anti-inflammatory properties of ginger essential oil are being shown to be the most active amongst all the essential oils tested.

Reference & Photo Credit:
http://www.ncbi.nlm.nih.gov/pubmed/24662935]

Study 5 – Gastroprotective Properties

In this study published in the *Journal of Basic and Clinical Physiology and Pharmacology*, the gastroprotective effects of ginger essential oil were examined, with the following results: "Turmeric (Curcuma longa) and ginger (Zingiber officianale) are widely used in Asian countries as traditional medicine and food ingredients. In the present study, we have evaluated the gastroprotective activity of turmeric essential oil (TEO) and ginger essential oil (GEO) in rats…Results suggest that TEO and GEO could reduce the gastric ulcer in rat stomach as seen from the ulcer index and histopathology of the stomach. Moreover, oxidative stress produced by ethanol was found to be significantly reduced by TEO and GEO."

The objective of this study was to evaluate the antiulcer effects of turmeric and ginger essential oils. In the study, rats with ethanol-induced ulcers were divided into groups to receive dosages of 100, 500 and 1000 mg/kg body weight, after which the effects of the essential oil treatments were assessed. Ginger essential oil was shown to inhibit the ulcer by 85.1%, by increasing the antioxidant enzymes and reducing the ethanol-induced lesions, including erosion, necrosis, and hemorrhage of the stomach wall. These results demonstrate ginger's gastroprotective activity and, moreover, indicate that the essential oil could potentially be used to relieve gastric ulcers.

Reference & Photo Credit:
http://www.ncbi.nlm.nih.gov/pubmed/24756059]

Study 6 – Acne & Cancer

In this study published by the *Molecules*, the lavender essential oil's effects on acne and cancer cells were examined, with the following results: "Ten essential oils, namely…ginger (Zingiber officinale Rosc., Zingiberaceae)…were tested for their antibacterial activities towards Propionibacterium acnes and in vitro toxicology against three human cancer cell lines…Time-kill dynamic procedures showed that thyme, cinnamon, rose, and lavender essential oils exhibited the strongest bactericidal activities at a concentration of 0.25% (v/v), and P. acnes was completely killed after 5 min…The cytotoxicity of 10 essential oils on human prostate carcinoma cell (PC-3) was significantly stronger than on human lung carcinoma (A549) and human breast cancer (MCF-7) cell lines."

This study tested ginger essential oil, along with other essential oils, against Propionibacterium acnes, the Gram-positive bacterium responsible for acne and other skin conditions. The study also looked at the essential oil's effects on lung cancer, breast cancer, and prostate cancer. Ginger essential oil demonstrated a 0.25 Minimum Inhibitory Concentration when it came to P. acnes. Ginger also showed cytotoxicity against the prostate and lung cancer cells. Although ginger essential oil was not the strongest of the oils tested, the results indicate that ginger can be effectively utilized in supporting the body's natural defenses against acne and prostate and lung cancer.

Reference
http://www.ncbi.nlm.nih.gov/pubmed/20657472]

http://www.mdpi.com/1420-3049/15/5/3200

Chapter 4 – The Ins & Outs of Essential Oils

Where do essential oils come from?

Plants and plant species naturally produce essential oils for various reasons, one being to draw pollinator insects to them, another being to repel invading organisms (bacteria, animals). Several chemical compounds compose each plant's essential oil, and the combination of these compounds are specific to each oil, which then instills in the oil its own unique properties. Essential oils can be harnessed from all sorts of plant components, including flowers, leaves, bark, fruit, roots, and resin. For instance, cinnamon oil is harnessed from bark, lemon oil from the peel, and lavender oil from lavender flowers. Certain plants can produce a few chemical variants of the same essential oil, which are acquired from different parts of the plant. Some of these parts produce a large amount of oil, while others produce just a smidgen. The oil's quality and potency depends upon many factors, including the subspecies of the plant, its soil conditions, the time of year and even the time of day you harvest it.

How are essential oils extracted?

Essential oils can be extracted from plants through various methods, including pressing, distillation, solvent and maceration. Let's take a brief look at each:

Pressing Method

Commonly used with citrus fruit, the pressing method extracts the oil through a technique which involves pushing the fruit peels through a press. Oily fruits and plants are best suited for this technique. Orange oil, for example, is extracted from orange skins through the pressing method.

Distillation Method

This technique harkens back to the days of old-timey moonshiners, as the same sort of method used to create strong liquor can be used to extract essential oils. Using a still, boiled water and plant materials will create steam which is then cooled by coils and condensed into a combination of water and oil. This combination doesn't mix, so the oil can then be extracted from it.

Solvent Method

Through a multi-step process, certain plant and flower oils can be extracted using alcohol and other solvents, which extort the essential oil from the plant materials.

Maceration Method

When a "carrier" or fixed oil or lard is mixed with the plant material and set out in the sun, over a period, the carrier oil is infused with the plant's essence. Heat sources, other than the sun, are often used to speed the process. Throughout the process, more plant material is added to produce a more potent oil.

7

How do you use essential oils?

Although some studies about the effectiveness of essential oils are conducted by small companies or even individuals, several them are conducted by the food and cosmetic industries. In general, the pharmaceutical industry shows next to no interest in herbal medicine, primarily because there are few options to patent such products. Being as such, the product's lack of profitability results in a lack of research funding. Regardless, the historical uses of essential oils tell us what we need to know: these oils have been effectively administered for centuries. The therapeutic qualifications of essential oils can be plotted in the survival of humans across cultures and generations.

Another reason that studies on essential oils have not resulted in much conclusive evidence as to their overall effectiveness is because definitive results are sometimes difficult to prove, as the quality of each batch of oil can vary for several reasons. One is that essential oils are impossible to standardize. As mentioned above, even the slightest variance in soil conditions and the time of harvesting – as well as innumerable other factors – will produce a different product quality and potency. In addition, essential oils are often obtained from various species of the same plant; Eucalyptus radiata and Eucalyptus globulus can both be used in the making of therapeutic-grade eucalyptus oil and, as a result, they may have slightly different properties and degrees of strength or effectiveness.

Just as there are several methods by which to extract essential oils, there are several methods to administer them therapeutically. The variety of chemical compounds in each essential oil means that their benefits and applications also vary across the board. Below are a few of these methods.

Topical Administration

Direct application of many essential oils works like a sponge, as skin sops up chemicals and other things (like sunlight, for instance). Topical application is best when you want to clear up an ailment on the skin's surface or in the underlying muscle tissue. When applying topically, you may either massage the oil into the skin or simply dab on the skin for therapeutic results. You might combine the essential oil with a carrier oil for topical use to dilute its potency. This is safer, as the oil is so concentrated. You may support your body's defenses against rash or muscle pain in this manner, but you should always test your patient for allergens before applying. Adverse effects are produced by natural chemicals as much as synthetic ones; poison ivy, for example.

To test for allergens, place a drop or two on your patient's inner forearm. If a rash develops within 12 to 24 hours, then the patient is allergic. In addition, phototoxicity – sun exposure resulting in an exacerbated burn – may be an issue when citrus oils are applied topically. So, one must proceed with caution when applying essential oils using this method.

Inhalation Therapy

Commonly known as "aromatherapy", this essential oil application is effective for inner ailments, like sore throat or cold. In a steaming bowl of distilled or sterilized water, add a few drops of essential oil and, with a towel over your head, bend over the bowl and inhale. The towel captures the vapors, making the technique even more effective. Essential oils can also be placed in a diffuser or potpourri throughout a room to produce somewhat diluted therapeutic effects.

Ingestion

When using this method, proceed with caution. Direct ingestion of essential oils must be monitored and applied in small doses that are diluted in a tablespoon or more of any carrier oil – olive oil, for example. If you are unsure of dosage amounts, make a tea with the relevant herb instead. Although the effects of this diluted use may be weaker, this application is a better alternative than an overdose of essential oils.

What are the general benefits of using essential oils?

Replacement for Prescription Drugs

One practical benefit for using essential oils is, of course, their substitutive nature. Many believe that they can replace Rx drugs, which is the ultimate reason to educate yourself on their application and to begin stockpiling your essential oil supply. Although it is our opinion that 100% pure essential oils that carry no harmful side effects are better to support the body and its functions, we recommend that you consult your physician before replacing your prescription or over-the-counter medications.

One of the potential threats of economic or social collapse is the lack of resources, and primarily the inability to procure prescription drugs. Being as such, finding suitable alternatives should be a priority when prepping for the worst.

Their portability is also a major bonus when it comes to survival prepping. The fact that these ultra-concentrated oils take up little-to-no space makes toting them to your shelter all the simpler should the need arise. And, because essential oils are highly concentrated, the application used in most procedures requires only a drop or two of oil, which means that tiny bottle will be long-lasting (example 15mL bottle contains approx. 250 drops).

Cheap, but Effective Alternative

Though money may be the last thing on your mind when it comes to prepping for a survival situation (money may even be obsolete in the event of social collapse), it is worth noting that the expense of essential oils pales in comparison to prescription drugs. In fact, whether you are forced to survive on essential oils due to a lack of prescription reserves, in some cases, you might consider substituting your prescriptions for these inexpensive alternatives regardless. Essential oils are a cheap, but equally effective alternative to prescription medicine.

No Expiration Date

Another benefit of essential oils is that they do not expire, neither do they have "proper storage" requirements. Many medicines and therapeutic products must be replaced every couple years, so this sets essential oils ahead of the pack when it comes to shelf life.

Versatility

Essential oils also offer great versatility. Apart from providing wellness benefits, essential oils can be repurposed for household and hygienic applications. For instance, if you're looking for something that might serve your dental hygiene needs in a time of crisis, thieves oil is your go-to essential oil. If you want to maintain your skin's wellness, frankincense and lavender will do the trick; the latter also serves as sunscreen, so you can prevent sun damage as well.

When it comes to the house or shelter, you can use essential oils to deodorize, which will come in handy in a disaster scenario where things might start to smell fishy due to lack of proper utilities and care. For example, after the 2011 tsunami and the subsequent nuclear reactor meltdown in Japan, a nurse named Risa Nakahira used essential oils to deodorize and sanitize putrid public bathrooms in overpopulated evacuation facilities. As relief workers searched for survivors, often wading through debris and decay, Nakahira also deodorized their boots and masks using essential oils. The possibilities of these natural oils are endless.

They are also versatile when it comes to the range of patients they're capable of supporting. The wellness of everyone from your great grandfather to your infant baby can be fortified with the aid of essential oils in the appropriate dosage. They even come in handy when supporting livestock or pets. From teething infants to dementia in the elderly, from teenagers with acne to dogs with urinary tract infections, essential oils can serve any patient with nearly any ailment.

8

Conclusion

Now that you know all about what ginger essential oil can do for you – where it originates, how it's extracted, its benefits and properties, and the different methods of administration – you can use it confidently to support the body's defenses against wellness issues and start to assemble a kit of essential oils for survival.

The various benefits of essential oils and their properties are countless. To build your own kit, first focus on acquiring the essential oils which may bear more relevance to your wellness issues or the potential wellness threats within your environment. When it comes to nausea and digestive issues, for instance, ginger essential oil will be one of your more crucial oils, due to its digestive properties.

Used as a supplement or as your go-to for inflammation, cardiovascular wellness, or respiratory issues, the application of ginger essential oil in medicine has survived for centuries and will survive centuries more. When it comes down to it, you don't need to rely on pharmaceuticals; essential oils, herbs, and plenty of other natural ingredients can be used to help support any number of wellness issues, whether ailment or injury.

Essential oils are essential to your survival in the case of viral outbreak, social collapse or natural disaster because, when the SHTF, your access to pharmaceuticals will likely either be limited or eliminated altogether. Alternatives to our modern-day standard will equate survival when no other option exists. And when it comes to a life-or-death situation, you can't let your wellness decline, no matter the state of the world.

DISCLAIMER AND/OR LEGAL NOTICES: Every effort has been made to accurately represent this book and it's potential. Results vary with every individual, and your results may or may not be different from those depicted. No promises, guarantees or warranties, whether stated or implied, have been made that you will produce any specific result from this book. Your efforts are individual and unique, and may vary from those shown. Your success depends on your efforts, background and motivation.

The material in this publication is provided for educational and informational purposes only and is not intended as medical advice. The information contained in this book should not be used to diagnose or treat any illness, metabolic disorder, disease or health problem. Always consult your physician or healthcare provider before beginning any nutrition or exercise program. Use of the programs, advice, and information contained in this book is at the sole choice and risk of the reader.